RESTLESS LEGS SYNDROME CURE HANDBOOK

A COMPLETE TO TREATMENT AND CURE OF RESTLESS LEGS SYNDROME

EMILEE WILLY

Table of Contents

CHAPTER ONE

What is the cause of restless legs?

RLS, also known as restless legs syndrome, is a neurological condition. Repetitive leg syndrome (RLS) is also known as Willis-Ekbom disease (WED) or RLS.

Leg pain and a strong desire to move your legs are both common symptoms of RLS. Relaxed or sleepy people are more likely to feel the urge to urinate.

For those who suffer from RLS, the greatest worry is that it will disrupt their sleep, resulting in excessive daytime sleepiness and exhaustion. Many health issues, including depression, can arise if you don't treat RLS and sleep deprivation.

According to the National Institute of Neurological Disorders and Stroke, RLS affects approximately 10% of the population in the United States. At any age, it can occur, but it's usually more severe in middle age or older. RLS is twice as common in women as it is in men.

RLS is associated with periodic limb movement sleep apnea (PLMAS), which affects at least 80% of patients (PLMS). While sleeping, the legs twitch or jerk. Every 15 to 40 seconds, it can happen, and it can go on all night. Sleep deprivation is another side effect of PLMS.

Medications can help manage the symptoms of RLS, but there is no cure.

What signs and symptoms are present?

An overwhelming urge to move your legs, especially when you're sitting still or lying down in bed, is the most common sign of RLS Your legs may also feel tingly, crawly, or as if they were being pulled in different directions. These sensations may be alleviated through physical activity.

If you have a mild case of RLS, you may not experience symptoms every night. These tics and twirls could be explained by feelings of anxiety, restlessness, or tension.

It's hard to ignore a more severe case of RLS. Going to the movies can be a nightmare because of it. Even a lengthy flight on an airplane can be taxing.

Because RLS symptoms are worse at night, people who suffer from it often have difficulty getting to sleep or staying asleep. Sleep deprivation and excessive daytime sleepiness can have negative effects on your physical and mental well-being.

There are some people who have symptoms on only one side of their body, but this is rare. It is possible for symptoms to come and go sporadically in people with mild cases. It's possible that RLS will affect not only your legs, but your arms and head as well. With age, the symptoms of RLS tend to deteriorate for the vast majority of sufferers.

The symptoms of RLS can be alleviated by moving around.

Pacing the floor or tossing and turning in bed could be examples of this. If you share a bed with someone, it's possible that you're causing them sleep disturbances as well.

RLS's etiology is frequently unknown. Genetic predisposition and environmental triggers are both possibilities.

Many RLS sufferers have a family history of the disorder. There are actually five gene variants that are linked to RLS. Symptoms typically appear before the age of 40 if the condition runs in the family.

Even if your blood tests show that your iron level is normal, there may be a link between RLS and low levels of iron in the brain.

Dopaminergic pathways in the brain have been implicated as a possible cause of RLS. Dopamine is also implicated in Parkinson's disease. So, it's possible that many people with Parkinson's also have restless legs syndrome (RLS). Both conditions are treated with the same drugs. These and other theories are currently the subject of research.

Caffeine and alcohol may exacerbate or trigger symptoms. Toxicology treatments may also be to blame.

- allergies

- nausea

- depression

- psychosis

CHAPTER TWO

There is no underlying cause of primary RLS. It is possible that RLS develops as a side effect of a more serious medical condition, such as diabetes or kidney disease. If this is the case, treating the underlying cause may be sufficient to alleviate RLS symptoms.

It is important to know what causes restless leg syndrome.

If you have a history of RLS, you may be at an increased risk of developing the condition.

However, it's not clear if any of these things are to blame for RLS.

• Gender: RLS is twice as common in women as it is in men.

• Age: RLS is more common and more severe after middle age, although it can occur at any age.

• Genetics: Having RLS is more likely if other members of your family suffer from it.

During pregnancy, RLS can be a problem for some women, especially in the third trimester. Within a few weeks of delivery, this problem is usually resolved.

RLS can be caused by a variety of chronic conditions, including diabetes, peripheral neuropathy, and kidney failure. RLS symptoms can be alleviated by treating the underlying condition.

Medicines such as antinausea, antipsychotic, antidepressant, and antihistamine medications can cause or exacerbate RLS symptoms.

People of Northern European descent are more likely to suffer from RLS than those of other ethnicities.

RLS can have a negative impact on both your physical and mental well-being. To a greater extent, people who suffer from RLS and chronic sleep deprivation are at risk for

coronary artery disease

• stroke

- diabetes

disease of the kidneys

- depression

- death at an early age

Restless leg syndrome is diagnosed

RLS cannot be confirmed or ruled out with a single test. Your description of symptoms will play a large role in determining the diagnosis.

incessant and sometimes irrational desire to move

At the beginning of the day, symptoms are mild to nonexistent, and they worsen at night.

When you try to unwind or sleep, you may experience sensory symptoms.

• When you move, your sensory symptoms go away.

Even if all of the requirements are met, you may still need a physical examination. Other neurological causes of your symptoms will be investigated by your doctor.

Don't forget to tell us if you take any prescription or over-the-counter drugs or nutritional supplements. Tell your doctor if you have any known long-term health conditions, as well

You can get a blood test to see if you have iron deficiencies or other abnormalities. An expert in sleep, neurology, or another field might be referred to you in the event that something other than RLS is at play.

Children who are unable to articulate their symptoms may have a more difficult time being diagnosed with RLS.

Symptoms may be reduced by using home remedies, which are unlikely to completely eliminate them. Finding the most effective remedies may require some experimentation.

Here are some ideas:

Reduce or eliminate the consumption of caffeine, alcohol, and tobacco.

• Make an effort to maintain a consistent sleep schedule, aiming for the same bedtime and wake-up time each day.

• Take a walk or swim every day to keep your heart rate up.

• In the evening, massage or stretch your calf muscles.

• Before going to bed, take a long hot bath.

A heating pad or ice pack can be helpful in relieving symptoms.

• Take up a new hobby, such as yoga or meditation.

Scheduling activities that require a lot of sitting, such as a car or plane ride, is best done in the morning.

Ask your doctor or nutritionist for advice on how to improve your diet if you have an iron or other nutritional deficiency.

Consult your physician before beginning a new supplement regimen. If you don't have a deficiency, taking certain supplements can be harmful.

Even if you are taking medication to control your RLS, you may benefit from these options.

Restless Legs Syndrome (RLS) Medication

RLS can't be cured, but medication can help alleviate its symptoms. Here are a few options:

CHAPTER THREE

Dopaminergic agonists (dopaminergic agents)

These drugs help to reduce the amount of movement in your legs.

This group of drugs includes:

and • pramipexole (Mirapex)

This is ropinirole (Requip)

the active ingredient in rotigotine (Neupro)

Lightheadedness and nausea are possible side effects. Over time, the effectiveness of these drugs may wane. RLS symptoms can be worsened in some people by daytime sleepiness and impulse control disorders.

Muscle relaxants and sleep aids (benzodiazepines)

These medications may not completely alleviate your symptoms, but they can help you relax and sleep better.

This group of drugs includes:

Clonazepam is a prescription sedative (Klonopin)

In the case of eszopiclone (Lunesta)

Temazepam is a prescription drug (Restoril)

zaleplon is one example of a word like this: (Sonata)

anxiolytics (Ambien)

Daytime drowsiness is one of the side effects.

Nootropics (opioids)

Pain and strange sensations can be lessened, and you can feel more relaxed, with the help of these drugs.

This group of drugs includes:

• codeine

In addition, oxycodone is available (Oxycontin)

• acetaminophen and hydrocodone together (Norco)

• oxycodone and acetaminophen in a single tablet (Percocet, Roxicet)

It is possible to experience dizziness and nausea as a side effect. Sleep apnoea sufferers should avoid using these products. These drugs have a high potential for abuse and dependence.

Anticonvulsants

Sensory disturbances are lessened by taking these medications:

The medication gabapentin (Neurontin)

The drug gabapentin enacarbil (Horizant)

pregabalin is a drug (Lyrica)

You may feel dizzy or tired as a result of the side effects.

You may have to try several medications before you find the one that works best for you. As your symptoms evolve, your doctor will make adjustments to the medication and dosage.

Pediatric restless leg syndrome

RLS can cause the same tingling and pulling sensations in children's legs as it does in adults. As for how to describe it, they may struggle. A "creepy crawly" sensation could be the best description.

RLS can cause children to have an overwhelming desire to move their legs. Symptoms are more common in children than in adults during the day.

Inability to get a good night's rest can have a negative impact on every aspect of one's life. If your child has RLS, you may notice that they are fidgety, irritable, or otherwise difficult to concentrate on. Disruptive or hyperactive, they may be labeled. RLS can be diagnosed and treated in order to address these issues and improve student performance at school.

Adult criteria must be met in order to diagnose RLS in children under the age of 12:

incessant and sometimes irrational desire to move

At night, the symptoms worsen.

When you try to unwind or sleep, the symptoms are exacerbated.

When you move around, the symptoms subside.

Additional requirements include a child's description of leg pain in their own words.

CHAPTER FOUR

There must be two of the following conditions:

- Old age is associated with a sleep disorder.

- RLS was inherited from a parent or sibling.

- A periodic limb movement index of five or more per hour of sleep is confirmed by a sleep study.

It is necessary to correct any nutritional deficiencies. Avoiding caffeine and developing good bedtime routines are essential for children with RLS.

Benzodiazepines, anticonvulsants, and dopaminergic medications may be prescribed.

For those who suffer from restless legs syndrome, here are some dietary guidelines

Those with RLS don't have to adhere to any specific dietary rules. Reviewing your diet to ensure that you are getting adequate amounts of vitamins and nutrients is a good idea, however. Reduce your intake of processed foods that are high in calories but have little or no nutritional value.

RLS can be caused by a lack of certain vitamins and minerals, which are deficient in some people. If this is the case, you may want to consider making dietary adjustments or supplementing your diet. In the end, it all comes down to what your tests reveal.

Try increasing your intake of iron-rich foods, such as meat, poultry, and seafood, if you are anemic.

- leafy greens such as spinach and kale

- peas

- Fruits and nut brittle

- beans

- red and pork meat

- Fish and shellfish

Some types of cereal, pasta, and bread that are fortified with iron

Because vitamin C aids in iron absorption, you may want to include these vitamin C-rich foods in your iron-rich diet:

citric acid, as well as citrus juices

There are a wide variety of fruits and vegetables that can be found here, including:

vegetables such as tomatoes and peppers

the greens of the cabbage family

Caffeine can be tricky. Some people may experience symptoms of RLS as a result of using it, but others report relief. Caffeine may help alleviate some of the symptoms you're experiencing.

Drinking alcohol can exacerbate the symptoms of RLS, as well as disrupt sleep. Avoid it at night, if at all possible.

The strange sensations you feel in your legs can be uncomfortable or even hurtful at times.. Sleep deprivation as a result of these signs and symptoms is a real problem for many people.

The dangers of sleep deprivation and exhaustion to your health and well-being cannot be overstated.

Restful sleep can be made more likely through the use of a variety of self-help techniques, including those listed below, as well as by consulting with your physician.

Take a closer look at your bedding. The old and lumpy ones may be time to get a new set. Comfortable sheets, blankets, and pajamas are also worth the investment.

• Ensure that your window coverings or curtains keep out unwanted light.

All electronic devices, including clocks and smartphones, should be kept out of the bedroom.

• De-clutter the bedroom.

• Avoid overheating by keeping the temperature of your bedroom on the cool side.

The first step is to establish a regular sleep schedule. Even on weekends, make an effort to maintain a consistent bedtime and rise time. It will help you get a good night's sleep.

Before going to bed, turn off all electronic devices at least an hour in advance.

- Just before going to sleep, take a hot bath or massage your legs.

Try sleeping with a pillow between your legs to see if it helps. It may prevent your nerves from constricting and causing symptoms, which could be beneficial.

Pregnancy and restless leg syndrome

In the last trimester of pregnancy, RLS symptoms may begin to emerge for the first time. Pregnant women may be up to three times more likely to suffer from RLS than the general population.

It's not clear why this is happening. Vitamin or mineral deficiencies, hormonal shifts, and nerve compression are all possibilities.

Leg cramps and insomnia are common side effects of pregnancy. There is a chance that these symptoms could be mistaken for RLS. Pregnant women with RLS should see their doctor if they are experiencing symptoms. You may need a blood test to determine if you are deficient in iron or other nutrients.

When it comes to the evening, try to avoid sitting for long periods of time.

• Even if it's just a short walk in the afternoon, try to get some exercise in each day.

Perform leg stretching exercises or a massage on your legs before you go to bed.

• If your legs are bothering you, try applying heat or cold to them.

Ensure that you get a regular amount of sleep.

Antihistamines, caffeine and smoking should be avoided.

• Ensure that your diet or prenatal vitamins are providing you with all the nutrients you require.

Pregnant women should not take some of the medications used to treat RLS.

Pregnancy-related RLS usually subsides on its own within a few weeks of delivery. If it doesn't, you should consult your physician about other options. If you're nursing, be sure to mention it.

Restless arm, restless body, and other related conditions are all examples of this syndrome.

CHAPTERT FIVE

"Restless leg" syndrome" is a term that refers to a condition that can also affect your arms, trunk, and head. Some people only have it on one side of their body, while others have it on both sides. It's still the same disease, despite the differences in appearance.

People with RLS also experience periodic limb movement while they sleep (PLMS). During sleep, the legs may twitch or jerk uncontrollably, which can last for the entire night.

Chronic conditions like diabetes and kidney failure can lead to a condition known as restless leg syndrome (RLS). Often, treating the underlying problem is the best option.

RLS is a common complication of Parkinson's disease. However, the vast majority of RLS sufferers do not develop Parkinson's disease. Both conditions can be treated with the same drugs.

Multiple sclerosis (MS) patients frequently experience sleep problems, including restless legs, limbs, and body. Muscle spasms and cramps are also a common occurrence in these individuals.. Chronic disease-related fatigue can also be exacerbated by medication used to treat it. Some people find relief with medication changes or natural solutions.

Pregnant women are more likely to suffer from RLS. After the baby is born, it usually goes away on its own.

Leg cramps or other strange sensations can strike anyone at any time. Get a proper diagnosis and treatment from your doctor if the symptoms are interfering with your sleep. Please mention any medical conditions you may have.

Restless legs syndrome (RLS) facts and statistics

Approximately 10% of the population suffers from RLS, according to the National Institutes of Health. One million children of school age are included in this total..

35 percent of RLS sufferers began experiencing symptoms

before the age of 20. By the age of ten, one out of every ten children is complaining of symptoms. With age, symptoms tend to get worse.

A woman is twice as likely as a man to develop breast cancer. Two or three times more likely than the general population are pregnant women.

People of Northern European descent are more likely to suffer from it than those of other ethnicities.

The use of certain antihistamines, antinausea, antidepressant, and antipsychotic medications can cause or worsen RLS symptoms.

A condition known as periodic limb movement of sleep (PLMS) affects about 80 percent of RLS sufferers (PLMS). PLMS is characterized by frequent, involuntary jerks or twitches of the legs, occurring every 15 to 40 seconds. People with PLMS are not likely to suffer from RLS.

RLS's underlying cause isn't always clear. Although 40% of

RLS sufferers have a family history of the condition, this is not always the case. Symptoms typically appear before the age of 40 if the condition runs in the family.

RLS is linked to five specific gene variants. About 75% of people with RLS have the BTBD9 gene change associated with an increased risk of developing RLS. About 65 percent of the population does not have RLS.

RLS cannot be cured. However, treatment with medication and a

change in lifestyle can alleviate
symptoms.

THE END